HCG COOKBOOK

MAIN COURSE - 60+ Easy to prepare home recipes for a balanced and healthy diet

TABLE OF CONTENTS

Introduction

HCG recipes for personal enjoyment but also for family enjoyment. You will love them for sure for how easy it is to prepare them.

BREAKFAST

BANANA PANCAKES

Serves: ***4***

Prep Time: ***10*** Minutes

Cook Time: ***20*** Minutes

Total Time: ***30*** Minutes

INGREDIENTS

- **1 cup whole wheat flour**
- **¼ tsp baking soda**
- **¼ tsp baking powder**
- **1 cup banana**
- **2 eggs**
- **1 cup milk**

DIRECTIONS

1. **In a bowl combine all ingredients together and mix well**
2. **In a skillet heat olive oil**
3. **Pour ¼ of the batter and cook each pancake for 1-2 minutes per side**
4. **When ready remove from heat and serve**

CRANBERRIES PANCAKES

Serves: ***4***

Prep Time: ***10*** Minutes

Cook Time: ***30*** Minutes

Total Time: ***40*** Minutes

INGREDIENTS

- **1 cup whole wheat flour**
- **¼ tsp baking soda**
- **¼ tsp baking powder**
- **1 cup cranberries**
- **2 eggs**
- **1 cup milk**

DIRECTIONS

1. **In a bowl combine all ingredients together and mix well**
2. **In a skillet heat olive oil**
3. **Pour ¼ of the batter and cook each pancake for 1-2 minutes per side**
4. **When ready remove from heat and serve**

DATE PANCAKES

Serves: *4*

Prep Time: *10* Minutes

Cook Time: *20* Minutes

Total Time: *30* Minutes

INGREDIENTS

- **1 cup whole wheat flour**
- **¼ tsp baking soda**
- **¼ tsp baking powder**
- **1 tablespoons date fruit**
- **2 eggs**
- **1 cup milk**

DIRECTIONS

1. **In a bowl combine all ingredients together and mix well**
2. **In a skillet heat olive oil**
3. **Pour ¼ of the batter and cook each pancake for 1-2 minutes per side**
4. **When ready remove from heat and serve**

STRAWBERRY PANCAKES

Serves: *4*

Prep Time: *10* Minutes

Cook Time: *20* Minutes

Total Time: *30* Minutes

INGREDIENTS

- **1 cup whole wheat flour**
- **¼ tsp baking soda**
- **¼ tsp baking powder**
- **1 cup strawberries**
- **2 eggs**
- **1 cup milk**

DIRECTIONS

1. **In a bowl combine all ingredients together and mix well**
2. **In a skillet heat olive oil**
3. **Pour ¼ of the batter and cook each pancake for 1-2 minutes per side**
4. **When ready remove from heat and serve**

JUJABE PANCAKES

Serves: *4*

Prep Time: *10* Minutes

Cook Time: *30* Minutes

Total Time: *40* Minutes

INGREDIENTS

- 1 cup whole wheat flour
- ¼ tsp baking soda
- ¼ tsp baking powder
- 2 eggs
- 1 cup milk
- 2 tablespoons jujabe fruit

DIRECTIONS

1. In a bowl combine all ingredients together and mix well
2. In a skillet heat olive oil
3. Pour ¼ of the batter and cook each pancake for 1-2 minutes per side
4. When ready remove from heat and serve

NECTARINE MUFFINS

Serves: *8-12*

Prep Time: ***10*** Minutes

Cook Time: ***20*** Minutes

Total Time: ***30*** Minutes

INGREDIENTS

- **2 eggs**
- **1 tablespoon olive oil**
- **1 cup milk**
- **2 cups whole wheat flour**
- **1 tsp baking soda**
- **¼ tsp baking soda**
- **1 cup nectarine**
- **1 tsp cinnamon**
- **¼ cup molasses**

DIRECTIONS

1. **In a bowl combine all wet ingredients**
2. **In another bowl combine all dry ingredients**
3. **Combine wet and dry ingredients together**
4. **Pour mixture into 8-12 prepared muffin cups, fill 2/3 of the cups**
5. **Bake for 18-20 minutes at 375 F, when ready remove and serve**

BANANA MUFFINS

Serves: *8-12*

Prep Time: ***10*** Minutes

Cook Time: ***20*** Minutes

Total Time: ***30*** Minutes

INGREDIENTS

- 2 eggs
- 1 tablespoon olive oil
- 1 cup milk
- 2 cups whole wheat flour
- 1 tsp baking soda
- ¼ tsp baking soda
- 1 tsp cinnamon
- 1 cup mashed banana

DIRECTIONS

1. In a bowl combine all wet ingredients
2. In another bowl combine all dry ingredients
3. Combine wet and dry ingredients together
4. Fold in mashed banana and mix well
5. Pour mixture into 8-12 prepared muffin cups, fill 2/3 of the cups
6. Bake for 18-20 minutes at 375 F, when ready remove and serve

PAPAYA MUFFINS

Serves: *8-12*

Prep Time: ***10*** Minutes

Cook Time: ***20*** Minutes

Total Time: ***30*** Minutes

INGREDIENTS

- 2 eggs
- 1 tablespoon olive oil
- 1 cup milk
- 2 cups whole wheat flour
- 1 tsp baking soda
- ¼ tsp baking soda
- 1 tsp cinnamon
- 1 cup papaya

DIRECTIONS

1. **In a bowl combine all wet ingredients**
2. **In another bowl combine all dry ingredients**
3. **Combine wet and dry ingredients together**
4. **Fold in papaya and mix well**
5. **Pour mixture into 8-12 prepared muffin cups, fill 2/3 of the cups**
6. **Bake for 18-20 minutes at 375 F, when ready remove and serve**

PEAR MUFFINS

Serves: *8-12*

Prep Time: *10* Minutes

Cook Time: *20* Minutes

Total Time: *30* Minutes

INGREDIENTS

- 2 eggs
- 1 tablespoon olive oil
- 1 cup milk
- 2 cups whole wheat flour
- 1 tsp baking soda
- ¼ tsp baking soda
- 1 tsp cinnamon
- 1 cup pear

DIRECTIONS

1. In a bowl combine all wet ingredients
2. In another bowl combine all dry ingredients
3. Combine wet and dry ingredients together
4. Fold in pear and mix well
5. Pour mixture into 8-12 prepared muffin cups, fill 2/3 of the cups
6. Bake for 18-20 minutes at 375 F

CHOCOLATE MUFFINS

Serves: *8-12*

Prep Time: *10* Minutes

Cook Time: *20* Minutes

Total Time: *30* Minutes

INGREDIENTS

- 2 eggs
- 1 tablespoon olive oil
- 1 cup milk
- 2 cups whole wheat flour
- 1 tsp baking soda
- ¼ tsp baking soda
- 1 tsp cinnamon
- 1 cup chocolate chips

DIRECTIONS

1. In a bowl combine all wet ingredients
2. In another bowl combine all dry ingredients
3. Combine wet and dry ingredients together
4. Fold in chocolate chips and mix well
5. Pour mixture into 8-12 prepared muffin cups, fill 2/3 of the cups
6. Bake for 18-20 minutes at 375 F, when ready remove and serve

PEACHES MUFFINS

Serves: *8-12*

Prep Time: ***10*** Minutes

Cook Time: ***20*** Minutes

Total Time: ***30*** Minutes

INGREDIENTS

- 2 eggs
- 1 tablespoon olive oil
- 1 cup milk
- 2 cups whole wheat flour
- 1 tsp baking soda
- ¼ tsp baking soda
- 1 tsp cinnamon
- 1 cup peaches

DIRECTIONS

1. In a bowl combine all wet ingredients
2. In another bowl combine all dry ingredients
3. Combine wet and dry ingredients together
4. Pour mixture into 8-12 prepared muffin cups, fill 2/3 of the cups
5. Bake for 18-20 minutes at 375 F
6. When ready remove from the oven and serve

ASPARAGUS OMELETTE

Serves: *1*

Prep Time: *5* Minutes

Cook Time: *10* Minutes

Total Time: *15* Minutes

INGREDIENTS

- **2 eggs**
- **¼ tsp salt**
- **¼ tsp black pepper**
- **1 tablespoon olive oil**
- **¼ cup cheese**
- **¼ tsp basil**
- **1 cup asparagus**

DIRECTIONS

1. **In a bowl combine all ingredients together and mix well**
2. **In a skillet heat olive oil and pour the egg mixture**
3. **Cook for 1-2 minutes per side**
4. **When ready remove omelette from the skillet and serve**

ZUCCHINI OMELETTE

Serves: *1*

Prep Time: *5* Minutes

Cook Time: *10* Minutes

Total Time: *15* Minutes

INGREDIENTS

- 2 eggs
- ¼ tsp salt
- ¼ tsp black pepper
- 1 tablespoon olive oil
- ¼ cup cheese
- ¼ tsp basil
- 1 cup zucchini

DIRECTIONS

1. In a bowl combine all ingredients together and mix well
2. In a skillet heat olive oil and pour the egg mixture
3. Cook for 1-2 minutes per side
4. When ready remove omelette from the skillet and serve

BROCCOLI OMELETTE

Serves: *1*

Prep Time: *5* Minutes

Cook Time: *10* Minutes

Total Time: *15* Minutes

INGREDIENTS

- 2 eggs
- ¼ tsp salt
- ¼ tsp black pepper
- 1 tablespoon olive oil
- ¼ cup cheese
- ¼ tsp basil
- 1 cup red onion
- 1 cup broccoli

DIRECTIONS

1. In a bowl combine all ingredients together and mix well
2. In a skillet heat olive oil and pour the egg mixture
3. Cook for 1-2 minutes per side
4. When ready remove omelette from the skillet and serve

BRUSSELS SPROUTS OMELETTE

Serves: *1*

Prep Time: *5* Minutes

Cook Time: *10* Minutes

Total Time: *15* Minutes

INGREDIENTS

- 2 eggs
- ¼ tsp salt
- ¼ tsp black pepper
- 1 tablespoon olive oil
- ¼ cup cheese
- ¼ tsp basil
- 1 cup brussels sprouts

DIRECTIONS

1. In a bowl combine all ingredients together and mix well
2. In a skillet heat olive oil and pour the egg mixture
3. Cook for 1-2 minutes per side
4. When ready remove omelette from the skillet and serve

ARUGULA OMELETTE

Serves: *1*

Prep Time: *5* Minutes

Cook Time: ***10*** Minutes

Total Time: ***15*** Minutes

INGREDIENTS

- **2 eggs**
- **¼ tsp salt**
- **¼ tsp black pepper**
- **1 tablespoon olive oil**
- **¼ cup cheese**
- **¼ tsp basil**
- **1 cup arugula**

DIRECTIONS

1. **In a bowl combine all ingredients together and mix well**
2. **In a skillet heat olive oil and pour the egg mixture**
3. **Cook for 1-2 minutes per side**
4. **When ready remove omelette from the skillet and serve**

CINNAMON & YOGHURT BREAKFAST BOWLS

Serves: *1-2*

Prep Time: *10* Minutes

Cook Time: *20* Minutes

Total Time: *30* Minutes

INGREDIENTS

- ¼ tsp cinnamon
- 6 figs
- 2 tablespoons orange juice
- 2 tablespoons honey
- ¼ lb. blackberries
- ½ lb. Greek yogurt
- 2 tablespoons granola

DIRECTIONS

1. In a bowl combine cinnamon, orange juice, honey and mix well
2. Add figs and mix well
3. Roast at 375 F for 18-20 minutes
4. When ready remove from the oven
5. Add remaining ingredients and mix well

OATMEAL WITH RAISINS

Serves: *1*

Prep Time: *5* Minutes

Cook Time: *5* Minutes

Total Time: ***10*** Minutes

INGREDIENTS

- **1 cup oats**
- **¼ cup coconut milk**
- **1 tablespoon raisins**
- **1 tablespoon apricots**
- **1 tablespoon almonds**

DIRECTIONS

1. **In a bowl combine all ingredients together**
2. **Refrigerate overnight**
3. **Serve in the morning**

EGG TACOS

Serves: 2

Prep Time: *10* Minutes

Cook Time: *10* Minutes

Total Time: *20* Minutes

INGREDIENTS

- 2 tablespoons olive oil
- 1 clove garlic
- 2 cups baby spinach
- 4 eggs
- 4 tortillas
- ¼ tsp cumin
- 1 can black beans

DIRECTIONS

1. In a skillet heat olive oil
2. Add garlic, beans and cook until golden brown
3. Add spinach, cumin, baby spinach and eggs
4. When ready pour mixture into prepared tortillas and serve

WALNUT OATMEAL

Serves: 2

Prep Time: *10* Minutes

Cook Time: *20* Minutes

Total Time: *30* Minutes

INGREDIENTS

- 2 cups oats
- 2 cups pineapple
- 1 cup walnuts
- 1 cup coconut milk
- 1 cup almond milk
- ¼ cup maple syrup
- 2 tablespoons honey
- ¼ tsp cinnamon
- 1 tsp vanilla extract

DIRECTIONS

1. In a bowl combine all ingredients together and mix well
2. Mix well and transfer mixture to a baking sheet
3. Press the mixture on the baking sheet and bake at 425 F for 18-20 minutes
4. When ready remove from the oven and serve

LUNCH

SIMPLE PIZZA RECIPE

Serves: *6-8*
Prep Time: ***10*** Minutes

Cook Time: *15* Minutes

Total Time: *25* Minutes

INGREDIENTS

- **1 pizza crust**
- **½ cup tomato sauce**
- **¼ black pepper**
- **1 cup pepperoni slices**
- **1 cup mozzarella cheese**
- **1 cup olives**

DIRECTIONS

1. **Spread tomato sauce on the pizza crust**
2. **Place all the toppings on the pizza crust**
3. **Bake the pizza at 425 F for 12-15 minutes**
4. **When ready remove pizza from the oven and serve**

ZUCCHINI PIZZA

Serves: *6-8*

Prep Time: ***10*** Minutes

Cook Time: *15* Minutes

Total Time: 25 Minutes

INGREDIENTS

- 1 pizza crust
- ½ cup tomato sauce
- ¼ black pepper
- 1 cup zucchini slices
- 1 cup mozzarella cheese
- 1 cup olives

DIRECTIONS

1. **Spread tomato sauce on the pizza crust**
2. **Place all the toppings on the pizza crust**
3. **Bake the pizza at 425 F for 12-15 minutes**
4. **When ready remove pizza from the oven and serve**

BUTTERNUT FRITATTA

Serves: 2

Prep Time: *10* Minutes

Cook Time: *20* Minutes

Total Time: *30* Minutes

INGREDIENTS

- **½ lb. butternut**
- **1 tablespoon olive oil**
- **½ red onion**
- **2 eggs**
- **¼ tsp salt**
- **2 oz. cheddar cheese**
- **1 garlic clove**
- **¼ tsp dill**

DIRECTIONS

1. **In a bowl whisk eggs with salt and cheese**
2. **In a frying pan heat olive oil and pour egg mixture**
3. **Add remaining ingredients and mix well**
4. **Serve when ready**

CORIANDER FRITATTA

Serves: 2

Prep Time: *10* Minutes

Cook Time: *20* Minutes

Total Time: *30* Minutes

INGREDIENTS

- **½ lb. spinach**
- **1 tablespoon olive oil**
- **½ red onion**
- **2 eggs**
- **¼ tsp salt**
- **2 oz. cheddar cheese**
- **1 garlic clove**
- **¼ tsp dill**
- **1 tablespoon coriander**

DIRECTIONS

1. **In a bowl whisk eggs with salt and cheese**
2. **In a frying pan heat olive oil and pour egg mixture**
3. **Add remaining ingredients and mix well**
4. **Serve when ready**

DILL FRITATTA

Serves: 2

Prep Time: *10* Minutes

Cook Time: *20* Minutes

Total Time: *30* Minutes

INGREDIENTS

- **1 tablespoon olive oil**
- **½ red onion**
- **¼ tsp salt**
- **2 eggs**
- **2 oz. cheddar cheese**
- **1 garlic clove**
- **1 tsp dill**

DIRECTIONS

1. **In a bowl whisk eggs with salt and cheese**
2. **In a frying pan heat olive oil and pour egg mixture**
3. **Add remaining ingredients and mix well**
4. **Serve when ready**

PROSCIUTTO FRITATTA

Serves: **2**

Prep Time: ***10*** Minutes

Cook Time: ***20*** Minutes

Total Time: ***30*** Minutes

INGREDIENTS

- **8-10 slices prosciutto**
- **1 tablespoon olive oil**
- **½ red onion**
- **¼ tsp salt**
- **2 eggs**
- **2 oz. parmesan cheese**
- **1 garlic clove**
- **¼ tsp dill**

DIRECTIONS

1. **In a bowl whisk eggs with salt and parmesan cheese**
2. **In a frying pan heat olive oil and pour egg mixture**
3. **Add remaining ingredients and mix well**
4. **When prosciutto and eggs are cooked remove from heat and serve**

PEA FRITATTA

Serves: 2

Prep Time: *10* Minutes

Cook Time: *20* Minutes

Total Time: *30* Minutes

INGREDIENTS

- ½ lb. pea
- 1 tablespoon olive oil
- ½ red onion
- ¼ tsp salt
- 2 oz. cheddar cheese
- 1 garlic clove
- 2 eggs
- ¼ tsp dill

DIRECTIONS

1. In a bowl whisk eggs with salt and cheese
2. In a frying pan heat olive oil and pour egg mixture
3. Add remaining ingredients and mix well
4. Serve when ready

BLACK BEAN BURGER

Serves: ***4***

Prep Time: ***10*** Minutes

Cook Time: ***30*** Minutes

Total Time: ***40*** Minutes

INGREDIENTS

- 2 cans black beans
- 2 eggs
- ¼ cup green pepper
- 2 tablespoons cilantro
- 1 tsp cumin
- ¼ tsp coriander
- ½ cup tortilla chips

DIRECTIONS

1. In a bowl combine beans, eggs, tortilla chips and seasoning
2. Mix well and form 4-5 patties
3. In a skillet heat oil and cook each burger for 4-5 minutes per side
4. When ready remove from heat and serve

CROCKPOT CHICKEN

Serves: ***4-6***
Prep Time: ***10*** Minutes

Cook Time: ***6*** Hours

Total Time: ***6*** Hours 10 Minutes

INGREDIENTS

- 2 chicken breasts
- 1 cup barley
- 2 cups chicken broth
- 1 bag mixed vegetables
- ¼ tsp onion
- ¼ tsp garlic powder
- 2 bay leaves
- 1 cup spinach

DIRECTIONS

1. Place all ingredients in a crock pot
2. Cover with a lid and cook on low until the vegetables are tender
3. When ready remove from the crockpot and serve

CHICKEN CUTLETS

Serves:	*4-6*	
Prep Time:	*10*	Minutes
Cook Time:	*20*	Minutes
Total Time:	*30*	Minutes

INGREDIENTS

- 2 lb. chicken breast
- ½ cup wheat flour
- 2 tablespoons butter
- 2 cups mushrooms
- ¼ cup red wine
- ¼ red onion

DIRECTIONS

1. Season the chicken and place the chicken in the bowl with the flour
2. In a skillet heat oil and fry the chicken for 4-5 minutes per side
3. When ready, remove from the skillet and set aside
4. In a pan add butter, mushrooms, onion and sauté until vegetables are soft
5. Add wine and simmer until the liquid has evaporated
6. Add the chicken back to the pan and cook until has thickened
7. Serve when ready

MUSHROOM SANDWICH

Serves: 2

Prep Time: *10* Minutes

Cook Time: *20* Minutes

Total Time: *30* Minutes

INGREDIENTS

- 1 lb. mushrooms
- 1 red onion
- ½ cup BBQ sauce
- 2 buns
- ¼ tsp pepper
- ¼ tsp salt
- 1 cup cabbage slaw

DIRECTIONS

1. In a bowl toss the mushrooms, onions, pepper, salt and spread the veggies on a baking sheet
2. Bake at 375 F for 12-15 minutes
3. Spread BBQ sauce on each bun
4. Place the roasted mushroom mixture on a bun
5. Top with the other bun and serve

COLESLAW

Serves: 2

Prep Time: 5 Minutes

Cook Time: 5 Minutes

Total Time: ***10*** Minutes

INGREDIENTS

- 2 carrots
- 2 purple carrots
- 1 cabbage
- ¼ red onion
- 1 bunch leaves
- 2 kale leaves
- 1 cup salad dressing

DIRECTIONS

1. In a bowl combine all ingredients together and mix well
2. Serve with dressing

CABBAGE SALAD

Serves: 2

Prep Time: 5 Minutes

Cook Time: 5 Minutes

Total Time: ***10*** Minutes

INGREDIENTS

- ½ cup bulgur
- 1 cabbage
- 1 red onion
- 1 cup parsley
- 1 tsp seasoning
- ¼ cup lemon juice

DIRECTIONS

1. **In a bowl combine all ingredients together and mix well**
2. **Serve with dressing**

CANTALOUPE SALAD

Serves: 2

Prep Time: 5 Minutes

Cook Time: 5 Minutes

Total Time: ***10*** Minutes

INGREDIENTS

- **1 cantaloupe**
- **1 cup olive oil**
- **¼ cup tarragon leaves**

DIRECTIONS

1. **In a bowl combine all ingredients together and mix well**
2. **Serve with dressing**

STEAKHOUSE SALAD

Serves: 2
Prep Time: *5* Minutes

Cook Time: *5* Minutes

Total Time: ***10*** Minutes

INGREDIENTS

- 2 garlic cloves
- 2 tablespoons mirin
- 2 tablespoons soy sauce
- 1 tablespoon olive oil
- 1 lb. steak
- 4 oz. snap peas
- 1 head lettuce
- 1 cucumber

DIRECTIONS

1. **In a bowl combine all ingredients together and mix well**
2. **Serve with dressing**

BUTTERMILK & JALAPENOS SALAD

Serves: 2

Prep Time: 5 Minutes

Cook Time: 5 Minutes

Total Time: *10* Minutes

INGREDIENTS

- **1 cabbage**
- **1 tablespoon olive oil**
- **1 cup buttermilk**
- **1 cup Greek yogurt**
- **¼ cup mayonnaise**
- **1 tablespoon lemon juice**
- **1 tablespoon chives**

DIRECTIONS

1. **In a bowl combine all ingredients together and mix well**
2. **Serve with dressing**

WATERMELON & JICAMA SALAD

Serves: 2

Prep Time: *5* Minutes

Cook Time: *5* Minutes

Total Time: ***10*** Minutes

INGREDIENTS

- 2 lb. watermelon
- ½ jicama
- 1 jalapeno
- 1 scallion
- ¼ cup cilantro

DIRECTIONS

1. **In a bowl combine all ingredients together and mix well**
2. **Serve with dressing**

SNAP PEA SALAD

Serves: 2

Prep Time: 5 Minutes

Cook Time: 5 Minutes

Total Time: *10* Minutes

INGREDIENTS

- 2 cups buttermilk
- 2 tablespoons lemon juice
- 1 garlic clove
- 6 oz. snap peas
- 2 tablespoon olive oil
- 1 tsp lemon zest

DIRECTIONS

1. **In a bowl combine all ingredients together and mix well**
2. **Serve with dressing**

CHICKPEAS SALAD

Serves: 2

Prep Time: 5 Minutes

Cook Time: 5 Minutes

Total Time: ***10*** Minutes

INGREDIENTS

- **1 can chickpeas**
- **2 tablespoon olive oil**
- **1 cooked chicken breast**
- **1 cup tomatoes**
- **1 cucumber**
- **1 cup feta cheese**
- **1 tsp oregano**

DIRECTIONS

1. **In a bowl combine all ingredients together and mix well**
2. **Serve with dressing**

RHUBARB SALAD

Serves: 2

Prep Time: 5 Minutes

Cook Time: 5 Minutes

Total Time: *10* Minutes

INGREDIENTS

- 2 rhubarb stalks
- 1 tsp salt
- 2 fennel bulbs
- 2 celery stalks
- ½ cup olive oil

DIRECTIONS

1. **In a bowl combine all ingredients together and mix well**
2. **Serve with dressing**

RICOTTA SALAD

Serves: 2

Prep Time: *5* Minutes

Cook Time: *5* Minutes

Total Time: ***10*** Minutes

INGREDIENTS

- **1 cantaloupe**
- **4 oz. snap peas**
- **4 oz. ricotta cheese**
- **2 tablespoons tarragon leaves**
- **2 tablespoons olive oil**

DIRECTIONS

1. **In a bowl combine all ingredients together and mix well**
2. **Serve with dressing**

DINNER

CHEESE MACARONI

Serves: *1*

Prep Time: *10* Minutes

Cook Time: *20* Minutes

Total Time: *30* Minutes

INGREDIENTS

- 1 lb. macaroni
- 1 cup cheddar cheese
- 1 cup Monterey Jack cheese
- 1 cup mozzarella cheese
- ¼ tsp salt
- ¼ tsp pepper

DIRECTIONS

1. In a pot bring water to a boil
2. Add pasta and cook until al dente
3. In a bowl combine all cheese together and add it to the pasta
4. When ready transfer to a bowl, add salt, pepper and serve

POTATO CASSEROLE

Serves: *2*

Prep Time: *10* Minutes

Cook Time: *20* Minutes

Total Time: *30* Minutes

INGREDIENTS

- 5-6 large potatoes
- ¼ cup sour cream
- ½ cup butter
- 5-6 bacon strips
- 1-2 cups mozzarella cheese
- ¼ cup heavy cream

DIRECTIONS

1. Place the potatoes in a pot with boiling water, cook until tender
2. Place the potatoes in a bowl, add sour cream, butter, cheese and mix well
3. In a baking dish place the bacon strips and cover with potato mixture
4. Add remaining mozzarella cheese on top
5. Bake at 325 F for 15-18 minutes or until the mozzarella is fully melted
6. When ready remove from the oven and serve

CHEESE STUFFED SHELLS

Serves: 2

Prep Time: *10* Minutes

Cook Time: *30* Minutes

Total Time: *40* Minutes

INGREDIENTS

- 2-3 cups macaroni
- 2 cups cream cheese
- 1 cup spaghetti sauce
- 1 cup onions
- 1 cup mozzarella cheese

DIRECTIONS

1. In a pot boil water and add shells
2. Cook for 12-15 minutes
3. In a baking dish add spaghetti sauce
4. In a bowl combine cream cheese, onion and set aside
5. Add cream cheese to the shells and place them into the baking dish
6. Bake at 325 F for 30 minutes or until golden brown
7. When ready remove from the oven and serve

POTATO SOUP

Serves: *4-6*

Prep Time: *10* Minutes

Cook Time: *50* Minutes

Total Time: *60* Minutes

INGREDIENTS

- 1 onion
- 2-3 carrots
- 2 tablespoons flour
- 5-6 large potatoes
- 2 cups milk
- 2 cups bouillon
- 1 cup water
- 2 cups milk
- 1 tsp salt
- 1 tsp pepper

DIRECTIONS

1. **In a saucepan melt butter and sauce carrots, garlic and onion for 4-5 minutes**
2. **Add flour, milk, potatoes, bouillon and cook for another 15-20 minutes**

3. **Add pepper and remaining ingredients and cook on low heat for 20-30 minutes**
4. **When ready remove from heat and serve**

CHICKEN ALFREDO

Serves: 2

Prep Time: *10* Minutes

Cook Time: *20* Minutes

Total Time: *30* Minutes

INGREDIENTS

- 2-3 chicken breasts
- 1 lb. rotini
- 1 cup parmesan cheese
- 1 cup olive oil
- 1 tsp salt
- 1 tsp black pepper
- 1 tsp parsley

DIRECTIONS

1. In a pot add the rotini and cook on low heat for 12-15 minutes
2. In a frying pan heat olive oil, add chicken, salt, parsley, and cook until the chicken is brown
3. Drain the rotini and place the rotini in pan with chicken
4. Cook for 2-3 minutes
5. When ready remove from heat and serve with parmesan cheese on top

BUTTERNUT SQUASH PIZZA

Serves: *4-6*

Prep Time: *10* Minutes

Cook Time: *15* Minutes

Total Time: *25* Minutes

INGREDIENTS

- 2 cups butternut squash
- ¼ tsp salt
- 1 pizza crust
- 5-6 tablespoons alfredo sauce
- 1 tsp olive oil
- 4-5 cups baby spinach
- 2-3 oz. goat cheese

DIRECTIONS

1. Place the pizza crust on a baking dish and spread the alfredo sauce
2. In a skillet sauté spinach and place it over the pizza crust
3. Add goat cheese, butternut squash, olive oil and salt
4. Bake pizza at 425 F for 8-10 minutes
5. When ready remove from the oven and serve

PENNE WITH ASPARAGUS

Serves: 2

Prep Time: *10* Minutes

Cook Time: *20* Minutes

Total Time: *30* Minutes

INGREDIENTS

- 6-7 oz. penne pasta
- 2-3 bacon slices
- ¼ cup red onion
- 2 cups asparagus
- 1 cup chicken broth
- 2-3 cups spinach leaves
- ¼ cup parmesan cheese

DIRECTIONS

1. Cook pasta until al dente
2. In a skillet cook bacon until crispy and set aside
3. In a pan add onion, asparagus, broth and cook on low heat for 5-10 minutes
4. Add spinach, cheese, pepper, pasta and cook for another 5-6 minutes
5. When ready sprinkle bacon and serve

NOODLE SOUP

Serves: ***4***

Prep Time: ***10*** Minutes

Cook Time: ***20*** Minutes

Total Time: ***30*** Minutes

INGREDIENTS

- **2-3 cups water**
- **1 can chicken broth**
- **1 tablespoon olive oil**
- **¼ red onion**
- **¼ cup celery**
- **¼ tsp salt**
- **¼ tsp black pepper**
- **5-6 oz. fusilli pasta**
- **2 cups chicken breast**
- **2 tablespoons parsley**

DIRECTIONS

1. **In a pot boil water with broth**
2. **In a saucepan heat oil, add carrot, pepper, celery, onion, salt and sauté until tender**
3. **Add broth mixture to the mixture and pasta**

4. Cook until al dente and stir in chicken breast, cook until chicken breast is tender
5. When ready remove from heat, stir in parsley and serve

TOMATO WRAP

Serves: *4*

Prep Time: *5* Minutes

Cook Time: *15* Minutes

Total Time: *20* Minutes

INGREDIENTS

- 1 cup corn
- 1 cup tomatoes
- 1 cup pickles
- 1 tablespoon olive oil
- 1 tablespoon mayonnaise
- 6-7 turkey slices
- 2-3 whole-wheat tortillas
- 1 cup romaine lettuce

DIRECTIONS

1. In a bowl combine tomatoes, pickles, olive oil, corn and set aside
2. Place the turkey slices over the tortillas and top with tomato mixture and mayonnaise
3. Roll and serve

THYME COD

Serves: 2

Prep Time: 5 Minutes

Cook Time: *15* Minutes

Total Time: *20* Minutes

INGREDIENTS

- **1 tablespoon olive oil**
- **½ red onion**
- **1 can tomatoes**
- **2-3 springs thyme**
- **2-3 cod fillets**

DIRECTIONS

1. **In a frying pan heat olive oil and sauté onion, stir in tomatoes, spring thyme and cook for 5-6 minutes**
2. **Add cod fillets, cover and cook for 5-6 minutes per side**
3. **When ready remove from heat and serve**

VEGGIE STIR-FRY

Serves: 2

Prep Time: *10* Minutes

Cook Time: *20* Minutes

Total Time: *30* Minutes

INGREDIENTS

- 1 tablespoon cornstarch
- 1 garlic clove
- ¼ cup olive oil
- ¼ head broccoli
- ¼ cup show peas
- ½ cup carrots
- ¼ cup green beans
- 1 tablespoon soy sauce
- ½ cup onion

DIRECTIONS

1. In a bowl combine garlic, olive oil, cornstarch and mix well
2. Add the rest of the ingredients and toss to coat
3. In a skillet cook vegetables mixture until tender
4. When ready transfer to a plate garnish with ginger and serve

SMOOTHIES

SUMMER SMOOTHIE

Serves: ***1***

Prep Time: ***5*** Minutes

Cook Time: ***5*** Minutes

Total Time: ***10*** Minutes

INGREDIENTS

- **½ cup Greek yogurt**
- **2 cups raspberries**
- **1 nectarine**
- **1 cup ice**

DIRECTIONS

1. **In a blender place all ingredients and blend until smooth**
2. **Pour smoothie in a glass and serve**

GREEN SMOOTHIE

Serves: *1*

Prep Time: *5* Minutes

Cook Time: *5* Minutes

Total Time: ***10*** Minutes

INGREDIENTS

- 1 cup almond milk
- 1 tablespoon honey
- 1 banana
- 2 cups spinach
- ¼ cucumber

DIRECTIONS

1. **In a blender place all ingredients and blend until smooth**
2. **Pour smoothie in a glass and serve**

TROPICAL SMOOTHIE

Serves: ***1***

Prep Time: *5* Minutes

Cook Time: *5* Minutes

Total Time: ***10*** Minutes

INGREDIENTS

- **1 banana**
- **1 pineapple**
- **1 cup mango**
- **1 cup almond milk**

DIRECTIONS

1. **In a blender place all ingredients and blend until smooth**
2. **Pour smoothie in a glass and serve**

BERRY SMOOTHIE

Serves: *1*
Prep Time: *5* Minutes

Cook Time: *5* Minutes

Total Time: ***10*** Minutes

INGREDIENTS

- **1 banana**
- **4 cups pineapple juice**
- **1 cup ice**
- **4 oz. blueberries**
- **4 oz. blackberries**
- **1 tablespoon honey**

DIRECTIONS

1. **In a blender place all ingredients and blend until smooth**
2. **Pour smoothie in a glass and serve**

CITRUS SMOOTHIE

Serves: *1*

Prep Time: *5* Minutes

Cook Time: *5* Minutes

Total Time: ***10*** Minutes

INGREDIENTS

- 1 cup carrot juice
- 1 banana
- 1 cup pineapple juice
- 1 cup ice

DIRECTIONS

1. **In a blender place all ingredients and blend until smooth**
2. **Pour smoothie in a glass and serve**

POMEGRANATE SMOOTHIE

Serves: *1*
Prep Time: *5* Minutes

Cook Time: *5* Minutes

Total Time: ***10*** Minutes

INGREDIENTS

- **1 cup pomegranate juice**
- **1 cup yogurt**
- **1 cup berries**
- **1 cup ice**
- **1 cinnamon**

DIRECTIONS

1. **In a blender place all ingredients and blend until smooth**
2. **Pour smoothie in a glass and serve**

PEANUT BUTTER SMOOTHIE

Serves: *1*
Prep Time: *5* Minutes

Cook Time: *5* Minutes

Total Time: ***10*** Minutes

INGREDIENTS

- **1 banana**
- **1 cup milk**
- **2 tablespoons peanut butter**
- **1 cup ice**

DIRECTIONS

1. **In a blender place all ingredients and blend until smooth**
2. **Pour smoothie in a glass and serve**

MANGO SMOOTHIE

Serves: *1*

Prep Time: *5* Minutes

Cook Time: *5* Minutes

Total Time: ***10*** Minutes

INGREDIENTS

- 1 cup orange juice
- ¼ cup vanilla yogurt
- 1 cup mango
- 1 carrot
- 1 cup ice

DIRECTIONS

1. **In a blender place all ingredients and blend until smooth**
2. **Pour smoothie in a glass and serve**

THANK YOU FOR READING THIS BOOK!